Welcome to your keto adventure.:)

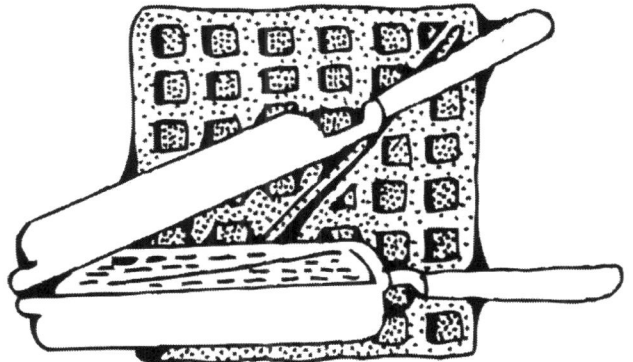

Contents

INTRODUCTION

WHAT IS A CHAFFLE?

It's simple, Egg + Cheese in a waffle iron = Chaffle.

A Chaffle is a Low-carb "Keto-Inspired" Waffle made with only 2 ingredients: Eggs and Cheese!
They are made with any type of grated cheese and can be made in many different flavors. You can add your favorite seasonings to your taste.

Before we begin, let's get a few things out of our way.

WHAT DO I USE TO COOK MY CHAFFLES?

Most people in the Keto world swear by the Dash "Mini" Waffle Iron. The reason a small one is better is because

1. you can make chaffle sandwiches that are crisp and just the right size,

2. Also, a regular/bigger chaffle maker makes the sandwich a little too thick.

3

CAN I USE A REGULAR WAFFLE IRON?

Yes, but it can take longer to cook your waffle crisp using a thick waffle iron. We suggest a mini waffle maker.

DO THEY TASTE EGGY?

The more ingredients you use in your chaffle preparation, the less likely they are to taste eggy.

You can use egg whites instead of the whole egg to make them taste less eggy.

HOW DO YOU SERVE CHAFFLES?

If the classic chaffle tastes a little too bland for your liking, experiment with various ingredients to suit your taste. Make chaffle sandwiches. Use as bread substitutes.

And coming to dessert and fruit chaffles, you can enjoy them as they are, or add cream as per your liking.

CAN I FREEZE MY CHAFFLES?

Yes. Just place them in a freezer bag separating each one with a piece of parchment paper, or just freeze them in small freezer bags, two per bag. You can use a microwave to defrost, or using an air fryer at 300F for 2-3 minutes when you're ready to eat.

Without further ado, let's get COOKING.

The "ORIGINAL" Chaffle Recipe

Ingredients

- 1 large egg
- 1/2 cup Cheddar
- 2 tsp of almond flour
- 1/2 tsp of baking soda

Instructions

- Preheat your waffle maker.
- Whisk together the egg, cheddar, almond flour, and baking soda in a bowl until well combined.
- Spray the waffle maker with cooking spray and pour the chaffle batter on top of the waffle maker. Close and let the waffle cook for 3 to 4 minutes.
- Take the waffle out of the waffle iron and enjoy.
- NOTE: The chaffle gets crispier as it cools.

Now that we have nailed our classic chaffle recipe, it's time to check out a few tips before we begin our adventure.

1. To properly and swiftly cook your chaffle, let the waffle maker get hot. This will prevent the mix from causing a sticky mess.

2. A bigger chaffle maker will take longer to crisply cook your chaffle. That's why we recommend a mini waffle maker.

3. In the waffle maker, put in a little cheese before you pour your chaffle mix, and then top it with a little more cheese before cooking. This will make them crispy.

4. Experiment with the amount of chaffle mix to pour into the waffle maker at any time. We'd rather you underfill rather than overfill and make a mess. When just starting out, you can use a silicon trivet underneath. This will make it easy to clean up.

5. Letting your chaffles cool for about 5 to 7 minutes can make them surprisingly crisp. Try with different levels of letting it cool to see for yourself.

6. Use egg whites if you find your recipes too eggy for your liking. Similarly, you can use mozzarella cheese to make them less cheesy.

7. You can freeze the chaffle. And even non-Keto citizens love them. So makes lots of them and spread the love.
   .

* * *

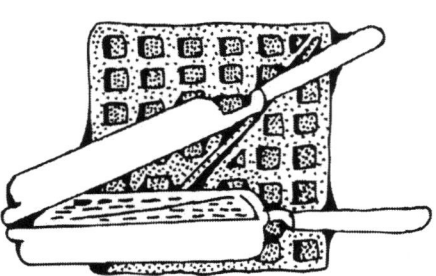

Chaffle Breakfast Ideas

* * *

LIGHT & CRISPY CHAFFLES

Ingredients

- 1 egg
- 1/3 cup cheddar
- 1/4 teaspoon baking powder
- 1/2 teaspoon ground flaxseed
- Shredded parmesan cheese on top and bottom.

Instructions

- Mix the ingredients together and cook in a mini waffle iron for 4-5 minutes until crispy.
- Once cool, enjoy your light and crisp Keto waffle.
- You can experiment with seasonings to the initial mixture depending on the mood of your taste buds.

CHAFFLE MCGRIDDLES

Ingredients

- 1 Egg
- 3/4 cup Shredded Mozzarella
- 1 Sausage Patty
- 1 Slice American Cheese
- 1 tbsp Sugar-Free Flavored Maple Syrup
- 1 tbsp Swerve or Monkfruit (or any sugar replacement of choice)

Instructions

- Pre-heat your Mini Waffle Maker
- Beat the egg into a small mixing bowl,
- Add shredded Mozzaerlla, Swerve/Monkfruit, Maple Syrup and mix until well combined.
- Place ~2 tbsp of the resulting egg mix onto the Dash Mini Waffle Maker, close lid and cook for 3 – 4 minutes. Repeat for as many waffles you are making.
- Meanwhile, follow cooking instructions for sausage patty and place cheese onto patty while still warm to melt.
- Assemble Chaffle McGriddle and enjoy!

CHAFFLE SANDWICH WITH BACON AND EGG

Ingredients

- 1 large egg
- 1/2 cup of shredded cheese
- thick-cut bacon
- fried egg
- sliced cheese

Instructions

- Preheat your waffle maker.
- In a small mixing bowl, mix together egg and shredded cheese. Stir until well combined.
- Pour one half of the waffle batter into the waffle maker. Cook for 3-4 minutes or until golden brown. Repeat with the second half of the batter.
- In a large pan over medium heat, cook the bacon until crispy.
- In the same skillet, in 1 tbsp of reserved bacon drippings, fry the egg over medium heat. Cook until desired doneness.
- Assemble the sandwich, and enjoy!

Keto BLT
Chaffle Sandwich

Ingredients

- 1/2 cup mozzarella, shredded
- 1 egg
- Bacon, pre-cooked
- Lettuce
- Tomato, sliced
- 1 tbs green onion, diced
- 1/2 tsp Italian seasoning
- 1 tbs mayo

Instructions

- Preheat the mini waffle maker
- In a small bowl, whip the egg.
- Add the cheese, seasonings, and onion. Mix it until it's well incorporated.
- Pour half the batter in the mini waffle maker and cook it for 4 minutes.
- **NOTE**: If you want a crunchy bread, add a tsp of shredded cheese to the mini waffle iron for 30 seconds before adding the batter. The extra cheese on the outside creates the best crust!
- After the first chaffle is complete, add the remaining batter to the mini waffle maker and

cook it for 4 minutes.

- Add the mayo, bacon, lettuce, and tomato to your sandwich.

Keto Stuffed Portobello Mushrooms

Note: although not technically a chaffle, we thought you'll love this keto stuffed mushroom recipe. Skip to next recipe if required.

Ingredients

- 4 Raw Portobello Mushroom caps, cleaned
- 4 oz. Cream Cheese, softened
- 3.8 oz. can Black Olives, sliced
- 8 Slices or 1 oz. each Provolone Cheese
- 1 oz. Pkg Fresh Basil
- 1 tsp Granulated Onion
- 1 tsp Granulated Garlic
- 1 tsp Smoked Salt (or pink)
- 1 tsp Smoked Paprika
- 1/2 tsp Black Pepper, fine
- 1 TBS Italian Herb Blend

Instructions

- Heat grill on med-high heat, or oven at 425.
- Clean mushroom caps, with stems removed. set them aside.
- In a small mixing bowl- Whisk softened cream

cheese with all seasonings.
- Prepare a grill pan or foil-lined baking sheet.
- Spread cream cheese mixture evenly among the 4 caps.
- Add about 1 oz. of sliced olives over top of the cream cheese.
- Then layer 2 slices or 1 oz. of cheese over the olives.
- Lightly salt/pepper a sprinkle, if you'd like.
- Cover loosely with foil.
- Grill or bake the caps for around 25-30 minutes, check for tenderness.
- Sprinkle some basil leaves over top and enjoy.

* * *

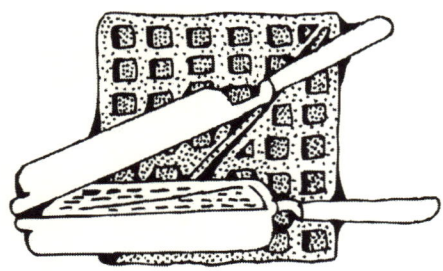

Veggie Loaded
Chaffles

* * *

Broccoli Cheese Chaffle

Ingredients

- 1 egg
- Garlic powder
- Cheddar cheese.
- Fresh chopped broccoli

Instructions

- In a bowl mix almond flour, cheddar cheese, egg and garlic powder. You can use a fork to mix everything.
- Add half the Broccoli and Cheese Chaffle batter to the Mini waffle maker at a time.
- Cook chaffle batter for about 4 minutes in the waffle.

- Let each chaffle sit for 1-2 minutes on a plate to cool slightly and firm up.
- Enjoy alone or dipping in sour cream or ranch dressing.

Zucchini Chaffles
or Zuffles

Ingredients

- 1 egg
- Small handful of shredded mozzarella
- 1 tablespoon parmesan
- 1 small zucchini, grated
- Basil and pepper to taste

Instructions

- Plug in the waffle maker to heat.
- Crack the egg and whisk for 20 seconds. Then add the rest of the ingredients and whisk again for 30 seconds until you get a smooth mix.
- Cook for about 4-5 minutes in the Waffle maker.
- Let the waffle cool and enjoy it crisp.

Cauliflower chaffle

Ingredients (Makes 4 mini chaffles, or two regular full-size chaffles.**)**

- 1 egg
- 1/2 cup shredded parmesan cheese
- 1/2 cup shredded mozzarella cheese or shredded mexican blend cheese
- 1/4 teaspoon Salt
- 1 cup riced cauliflower
- 1/4 teaspoon Garlic Powder
- 1/4 teaspoon Ground Black Pepper
- 1/2 teaspoon Italian Seasoning

Instructions

- Add all ingredients into a blender.
- Sprinkle 1/8 cup parmesan cheese into the waffle maker. Make sure to cover the bottom of the waffle iron.
- Fill the waffle maker with the cauliflower mixture.
- Add another sprinkle of parmesan cheese on top of the mixture.
- Cook for 4-5 minutes, or until crispy.

JICAMA LOADED BAKED POTATO CHAFFLE

Ingredients

- 1 cup cheese of choice
- 2 eggs, whisked
- 1 large jicama root
- 1/2 medium onion, minced
- Salt and Pepper
- 2 garlic cloves, pressed

Instructions

- Peel jicama and shred in food processor
- In a large colander, place the shredded jicama, and sprinkle with 1-2 tsp of salt. Mix well and allow to drain.
- Squeeze out as much liquid as possible.
- Microwave for 5-8 minutes
- Mix all ingredients together
- Sprinkle a little cheese on waffle iron, then add 1/3 of the mixture, and sprinkle a little more cheese on top of the mixture.
- Cook for 5 minutes. Flip and cook 2 more.
- Top with a dollop of sour cream, bacon pieces, cheese, and chives.

Spinach and Artichoke Chicken Chaffle

Ingredients

- egg
- 1/3 cup shredded mozzarella
- 1 ounce cream cheese
- 1/4 tsp garlic powder
- 1/3 cup cooked diced chicken
- 1/3 cup cooked spinach chopped
- 1/3 marinated artichokes chopped

Instructions

- Heat up your mini waffle maker.
- In a small bowl mix the egg, garlic powder, cream cheese and Mozzarella Cheese.
- Add the spinach, artichoke and chicken and mix well.
- Add 1/3 of the batter into your mini waffle maker and cook for 4 minutes. If they are still a bit uncooked leave it cooking for another 2 minutes. Then cook the rest of the batter to make a second chaffle and then cook the third chaffle.
- After cooking remove from the pan and let it sit for 2 minutes.
- Dip in ranch dressing, sour cream or enjoy alone.

* * *

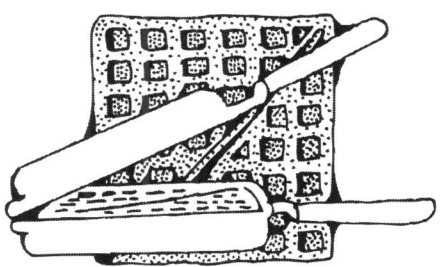

Fruit Chaffles

* * *

Strawberry
Shortcake Chaffle

Ingredients

- 1 egg
- 1/4 cup mozzarella cheese
- 1 tbs cream cheese
- 1/4 tsp baking powder
- 2 strawberries sliced
- 1 tsp strawberry extract

Instructions

- Preheat waffle maker.
- In a small bowl, whip the egg. Then, add the remaining ingredients.
- Spray the waffle maker with non stick cooking spray.
- Divide mixture in half.
- Cook half the mixture for about 4 minutes or until golden brown. Repeat with the second half.
- Top with simple whipped cream and strawberries.

Banana Nut Chaffle

Ingredients

- 1 egg
- 1 tbs cream cheese. softened and room temp
- 1/2 cup mozzarella cheese
- 1 tbs Monkfruit
- 1/4 tsp vanilla extract
- 1/4 tsp banana extract
- 1 tbs sugar free cheesecake pudding (dirty keto, so optional)
- Optional Toppings: Sugar free caramel sauce, Pecans (or any favorite nuts)

Instructions

- Preheat your waffle maker.
- In a small bowl, whip the egg.
- Add the remaining ingredients to the egg mixture and mix it until it's well incorporated.
- Add half the batter to the waffle maker and cook it for a around 4 minutes until it's golden brown.
- Remove the finished chaffle and add the other half of the batter to cook the other chaffle.
- Top with your optional ingredients and serve warm.

Blueberry Chaffle

Ingredients

- 1 egg
- 3 tablespoons almond flour
- 1 tablespoon cream cheese
- 1/4 teaspoon baking powder
- 5 or 6 blueberries
- 1 teaspoon blueberry extract, (optional)

Instructions

- Preheat waffle maker. Then, spray some nonstick cooking spray.
- In a small bowl, whip the egg.
- Add the remaining ingredients.
- Divide mixture in half.
- Cook half the mixture for about 3 to 4 minutes or until golden brown.
- Repeat with the remaining half.
- Allow the chaffles to cool. Top with these possible options: dust with monkfruit, more blueberries, whipped cream, frosting, or just eat it plain.

Pumpkin Chaffle

Ingredients

- 2 large eggs
- 1 cup finely shredded mozzarella cheese
- 1/4 cup pumpkin puree
- 2 teaspoons pumpkin pie spice
- 2 teaspoons coconut flour
- 1/2 teaspoon vanilla

Instructions

- Plug in waffle maker to preheat. Spray with non-stick spray.
- Add the eggs, pumpkin puree, pumpkin pie spice, coconut flour, and vanilla to a small bowl and whisk well to combine.
- Stir in the cheese.
- Spoon 1/4 of the batter into the hot waffle iron and smooth the batter out to the edges of the waffle iron.
- Close the iron and cook for 3 minutes.
- Remove the waffle and set aside. Repeat with remaining batter.
- Serve hot with butter and sugar free syrup.

Key lime Chaffle

Ingredients (for 3 to 4 mini chaffles)

Chaffle ingredients

- 1 egg
- 2 tsp cream cheese room temp
- 1 tsp powdered sweetener swerve or monkfruit
- 1/2 tsp baking powder
- 1/2 tsp lime zest
- 1/4 cup Almond flour
- 1/2 tsp lime extract or 1 tsp fresh squeezed lime juice
- Pinch of salt

Cream Cheese Lime Frosting ingredients

- 4 oz cream cheese softened
- 4 tbs butter
- 2 tsp powdered sweetener swerve or monkfruit
- 1 tsp lime extract
- 1/2 tsp lime zest

Instructions

- Preheat the mini waffle iron.
- In a blender add all the chaffle ingredients and

blend on high until the mixture is smooth and creamy.

- Cook each chaffle about 3 to 4 minutes until it's golden brown.
- While the chaffles are cooking, prepare the frosting.
- In a small bowl, combine all the ingredients for the frosting and mix until smooth.
- Allow the chaffles to completely cool before frosting them.

* * *

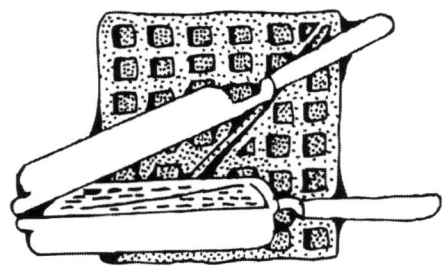

Italian-style
Chaffles

* * *

Pizza Chaffle

Ingredients

- 1 egg
- 1/2 cup mozzarella cheese shredded
- pinch of Italian seasoning
- 1 tbsp of zero sugar pizza sauce
- for topping, shredded cheese and pepperoni (or any topping of choice)

Instructions

- Preheat your waffle maker.
- In a small bowl, whip the egg and seasonings together.
- Mix in the shredded cheese.
- Add a tsp of shredded cheese to the preheated waffle maker and let it cook for about 30 seconds. This will help to create a more crisp crust.
- Add half the mixture to the waffle maker and cook it for about 4 minutes until it's golden brown and slightly crispy.
- Once done, remove the cooked waffle.
- Add the remaining mixture to the waffle maker to prepare the second chaffle.
- Top with a tablespoon of pizza sauce, shredded cheese, and pepperoni. Microwave it on high for

about 20 seconds and enjoy.

Cheesy garlic chaffle bread

Ingredients

1. 1 egg
2. 1/2 cup mozzarella cheese, shredded
3. 1 tbsp parmesan cheese
4. 3/4 tsp coconut flour
5. 1/4 tsp baking powder
6. 1/8 tsp Italian Seasoning
7. pinch of salt
8. 1 tbsp butter, melted
9. 1/4 tsp garlic powder
10. 1/2 cup mozzarella cheese, shredded
11. 1/4 tsp basil seasoning

Instructions

- Preheat oven to 400 degrees. Plug the Dash Mini Waffle Maker in the wall and allow to get hot. Lightly grease waffle maker.
- Combine the first 7 ingredients (NUMBERED above) in a small bowl and stir well to combine.
- Spoon half of the batter on the waffle maker and close. Cook for 3-4 minutes or until golden brown.
- Remove the chaffle bread carefully from the Dash

Mini Waffle Maker, then repeat for the rest of the batter.

- In a small bowl, melt the butter and add garlic powder.
- Cut each chaffle in half (or thirds) and place on a baking sheet then brush the tops with the garlic butter mixture.
- Top with mozzarella cheese and pop in the oven for 4 -5 minutes.
- Turn oven to broil and move baking pan to the top shelf for 1-2 minutes so that the cheese begins to bubble and turn golden brown. (NOTE: BE careful as it can burn quickly on broil.)
- Remove from oven and sprinkle basil seasoning on top. Enjoy.

Parmesan garlic chaffles

Ingredients

- 1/2 cup shredded mozzarella cheese
- 1 whole egg, beaten
- 1/4 cup grated Parmesan cheese
- 1 teaspoon Italian Seasoning
- 1/4 teaspoon garlic powder

Instructions

- Start pre-heating your waffle maker, and let's start preparing the batter.
- Add in all the ingredients, except for the mozzarella cheese to a bowl and whisk. Add in the cheese and mix until well combined.
- Spray your waffle plates with nonstick spray and add half the batter to the center. Close the lid and cook for 3-5 minutes, depending on how crispy you want your Chaffles.
- Serve with a drizzle of olive oil, grated Parmesan cheese and fresh chopped parsley or basil.

Savory Herb Chaffle

Ingredients

- 1 large egg
- 1/4 cup Mozzarella
- 1/4 cup parmesan
- 1/2 Tbsp butter melted
- 1 tsp herb blend seasoning
- 1/2 tsp salt

Instructions

- Heat your mini waffle maker
- Holding back a small amount of Mozzarella, mix everything together making sure egg is well incorporated.
- Put a small amount of Mozzarella onto the bottom of the waffle maker, pour 1/4 mixture on top if the cheese then put more Mozzarella on top.
- Cook for 4-5 minutes.
- Let it cool and then enjoy your savory herb chaffle

* * *

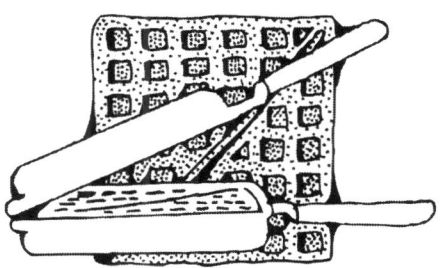

Keto Dessert Chaffles

* * *

Oreo Chaffle

Ingredients

- 1 egg1
- 1 tbs black cocoa
- 1 tbs monkfruit or keto-approved sweetener
- 1/4 tsp baking powder
- 2 tbs cream cheese
- 1 tbs mayonnaise
- 1/4 tsp instant coffee powder
- pinch salt
- 1 tsp vanilla

Frosting ingredients

- 2 Tbs monkfruit confectioners
- 2 Tbs cream cheese
- /4 tsp clear vanilla

Instructions

- Preheat you waffle maker.
- In a small bowl, whip up the egg.
- Add the remaining ingredients and mix well until the batter is smooth and creamy.
- Divide the batter into 3 and pour each in a mini waffle maker and cook it for around 3 minutes.

- In a separate small bowl, add the sweetener, cream cheese, and vanilla. Mix the frosting until everything is well incorporated.
- After it has completely cooled down to room temperature, spread the frosting on the waffle cake.

Vanilla Twinkie Chaffle

Ingredients (serves 4)

- 2 large eggs
- 2 tablespoons butter, melted (cooled)
- 2 ounces cream cheese, softened
- 1 teaspoon vanilla extract
- 1/4 cup almond flour
- 1 teaspoon baking powder
- 2 tablespoons coconut flour
- 1/4 cup Lakanto Confectioners
- Pinch of pink salt
- 1/2 teaspoon Vanilla Cupcake extract (optional)

Instructions

- Preheat your corndog maker.
- Melt the butter and let it cool a minute.
- Whisk the eggs into the butter until creamy.
- Add vanilla, extract, sweetener, salt and then blend well.
- Add Almond flour, coconut flour, and baking powder and blend until well incorporated.
- Add ~2 tbs batter to each well and spread across evenly.
- Cook for 4 minutes.
- Remove, let it cool, and enjoy.

Choco Chip Chaffle

Ingredients

- 1 large egg
- 1 teaspoon coconut flour
- 1 teaspoon monkfruit sweetener
- 1/2 teaspoon vanilla extract
- 1/2 cup finely
- shredded mozzarella
- 2 tablespoons sugar-free chocolate chips

Instructions

- Preheat your waffle maker..
- Add the egg, coconut flour, sweetener, and vanilla to a small bowl and whisk together with a fork.
- Stir in the shredded cheese.
- Spoon half of the batter into the waffle iron and dot with half of the chocolate chips. Spread a bit of batter over each chocolate chip.
- Close the waffle iron and cook for 3-4 minutes or until as crisp as you'd like.
- Repeat with remaining batter.
- Serve hot with whipped cream or low carb ice cream.

Keto Churro Chaffle

Ingredients

- 1 egg
- 1/2 cup mozzarella cheese shredded
- 2 tbsp Swerve/ monkfruit Sweetener
- 1/2 teaspoon cinnamon

Instructions

- Preheat your mini waffle maker.
- In a small bowl, whip the egg with a fork.
- Add the shredded cheese to the egg mixture, and mix lightly.
- Place half of the egg mixture in the waffle maker and cook it until it's golden brown (for about 3-4 minutes)
- While the chaffle is cooking, add the sweetener of choice and cinnamon in a separate small bowl.
- Once the Chaffle is done, cut it into slices while it's still hot and add it to the cinnamon mixture. It soaks up more of the mixture when it's still hot!
- Serve warm and enjoy.

Cinnamon Apple Chaffle

Ingredients

Chaffle ingredients

- 1/2 teaspoon monk fruit sweetener
- 3 large eggs
- 1 teaspoon baking powder
- 1/4 cup granny smith apple, skinned + diced
- 2 tablespoon coconut flour
- 2 teaspoons cinnamon
- 3/4 cup mozzarella cheese, shredded
- 1/4 cup mild cheddar cheese, shredded

Vanilla Bean Sauce ingredients

- 1 egg yolk
- 1/2 teaspoon monk fruit sweetener
- 1/2 teaspoon vanilla extract
- 2 ounces cream cheese, softened
- 1 cup whipping cream
- 1 tablespoon ghee (or butter)
- Vanilla bean, whole

Instructions

Vanilla Bean Sauce:

- In a medium saucepan, add heavy whipping cream, ghee, and vanilla bean.
- Heat over medium high heat until just starting to boil, then add sweetener and lower heat and simmer for 10 minutes. Remove vanilla bean and scrape remaining vanilla seeds into whipping cream, then discard bean.
- Remove from heat and add in egg yolk while whisking vigorously.
- Stir in cream cheese until melted.
- Put vanilla sauce in heat safe container and place in fridge to cool.

Apple Chaffle:

- Preheat waffle maker and spray with low carb non-stick spray.
- In a large mixing bowl, add egg and beat until frothy.
- Mix vanilla and cheese and beat until well combined.
- In a small mixing bowl, whisk together flour, baking powder, sweetener, and cinnamon.
- Add dry ingredients to egg mixture and mix until just combined.
- Gently top the mixture with diced apples.
- Pour batter into waffle maker on medium, high heat and cook until for about 4 minutes or starting to brown on the outside.
- Let the chaffle cool slightly, and then top with vanilla sauce.

Made in the USA
Coppell, TX
18 December 2019

13284321R00028